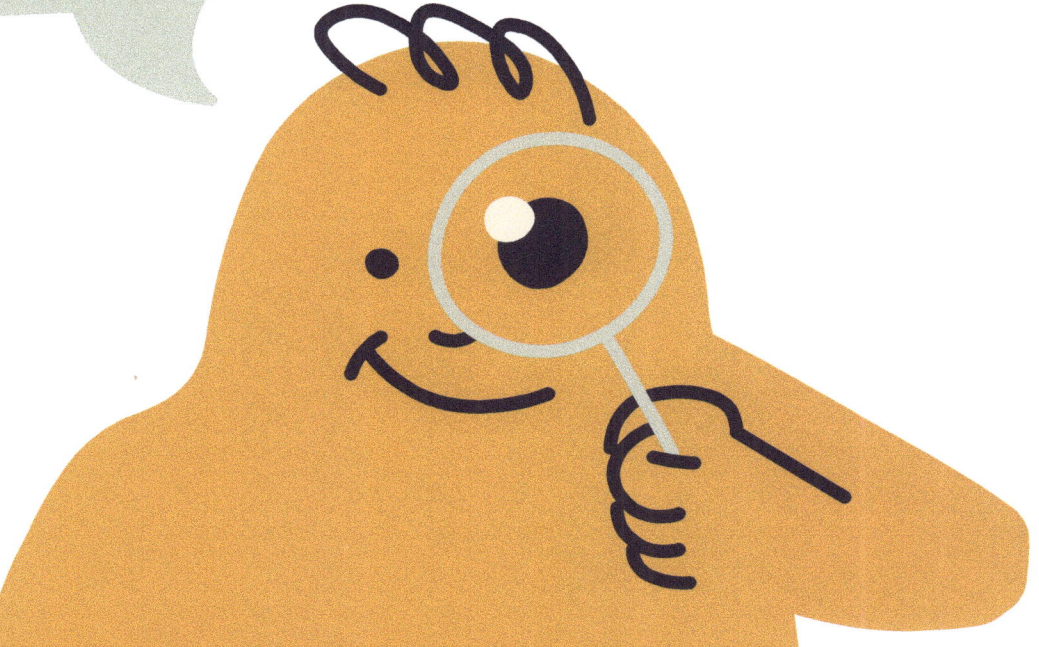

Looking for something to do? Check out the activities in the back of the book!

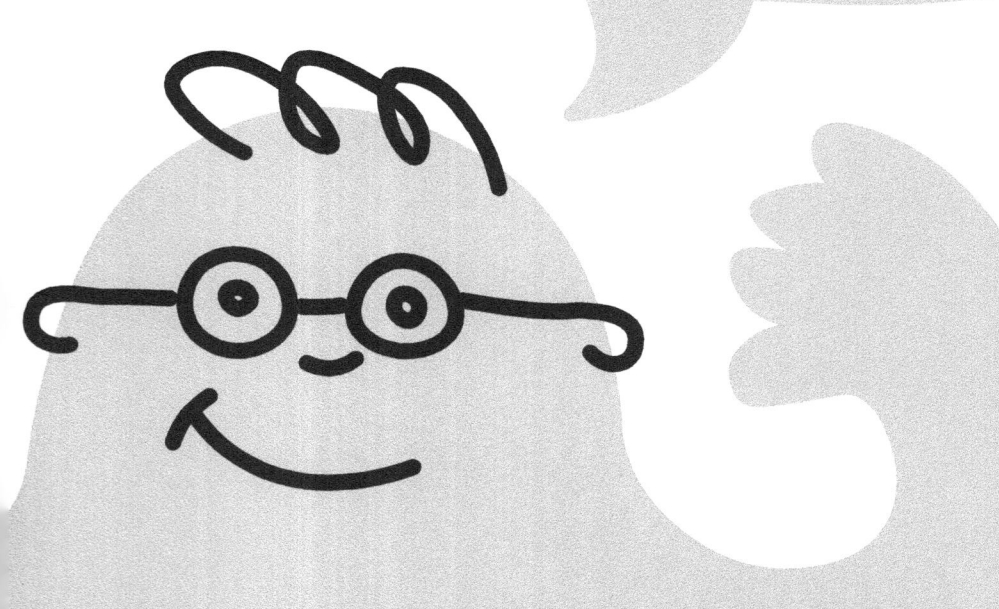

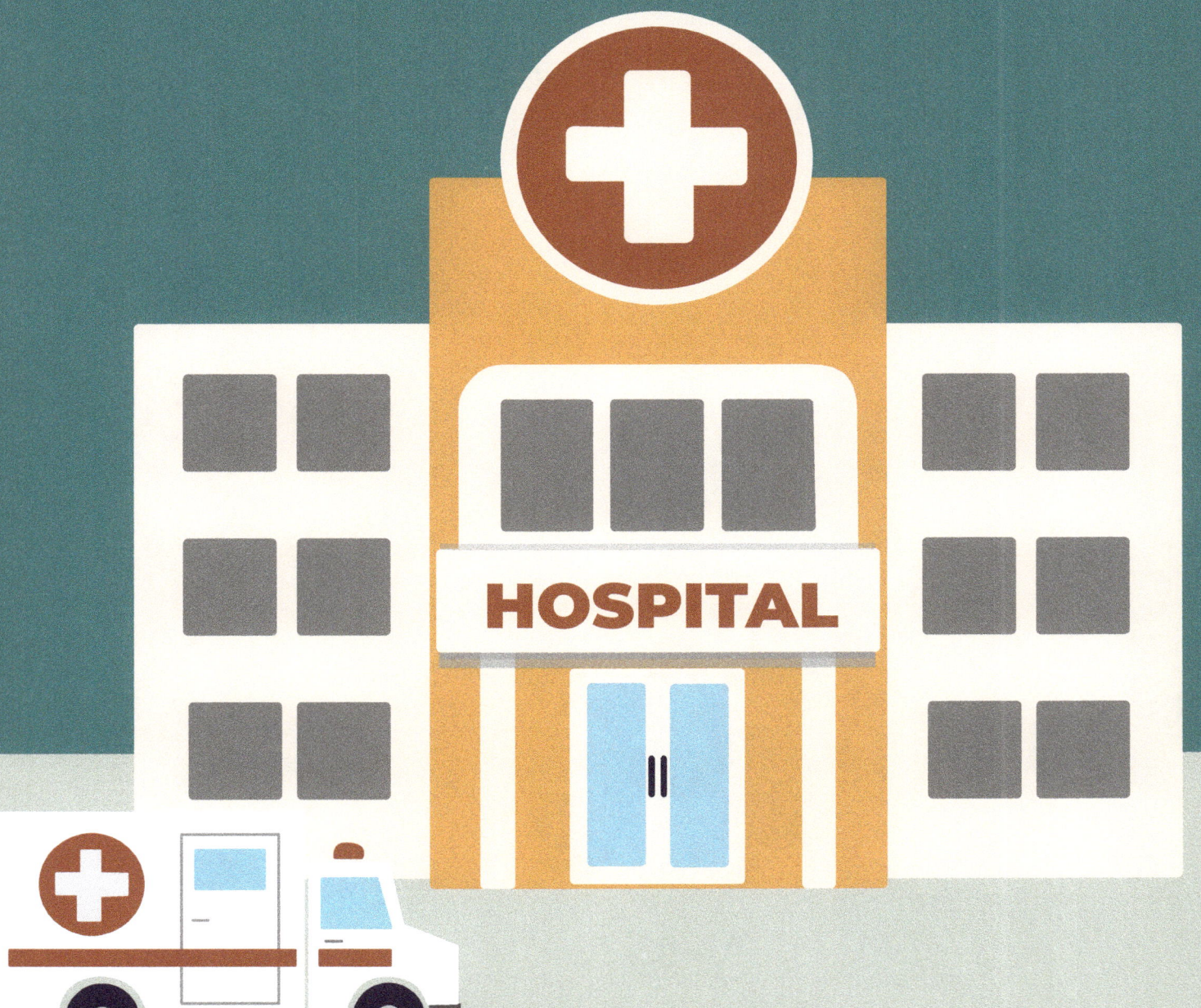

A hospital is a safe place where kids have a team of people to take care of them.

When a kid's body is hurt or sick, the team's job is to help them heal and feel better.

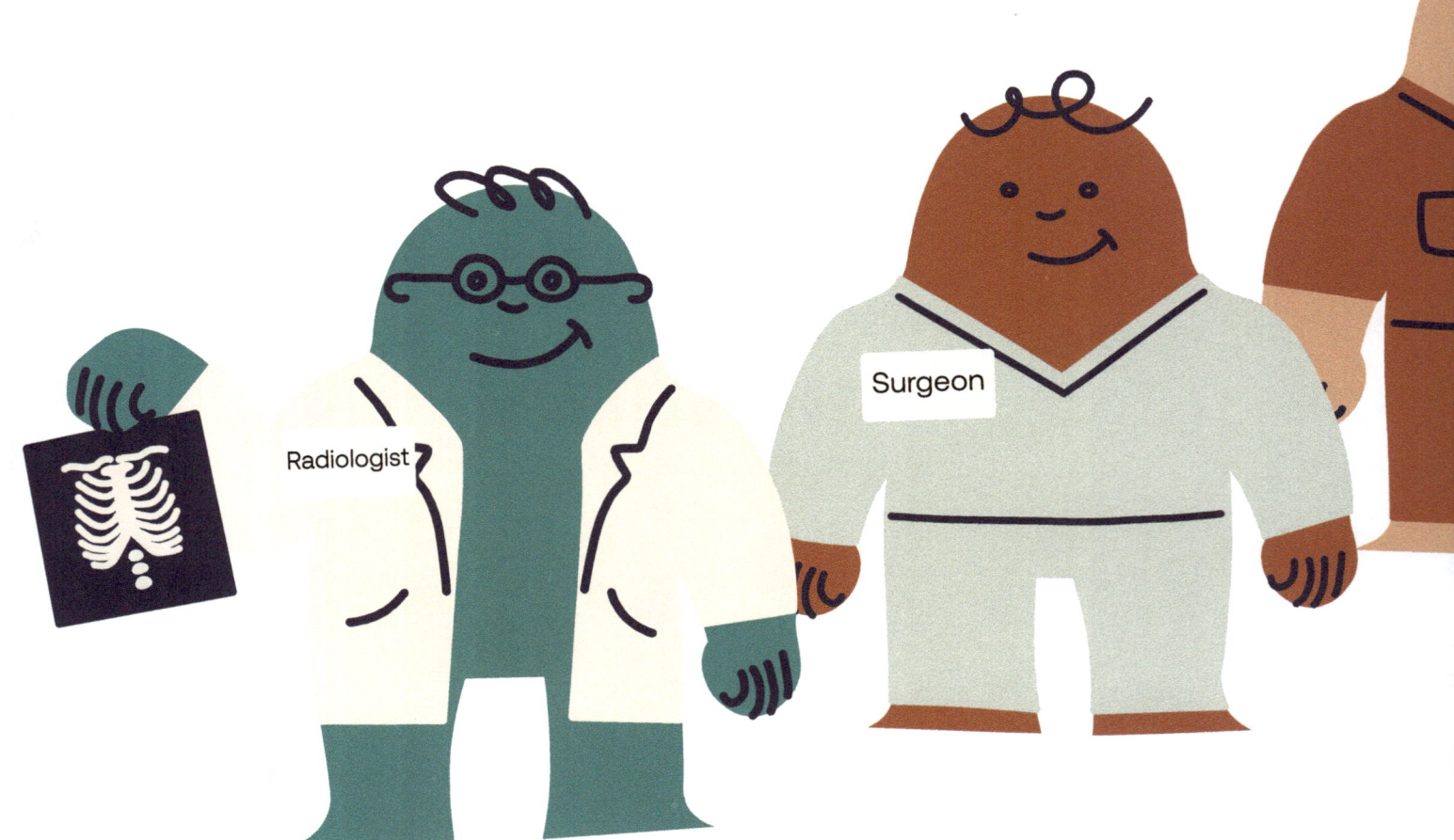

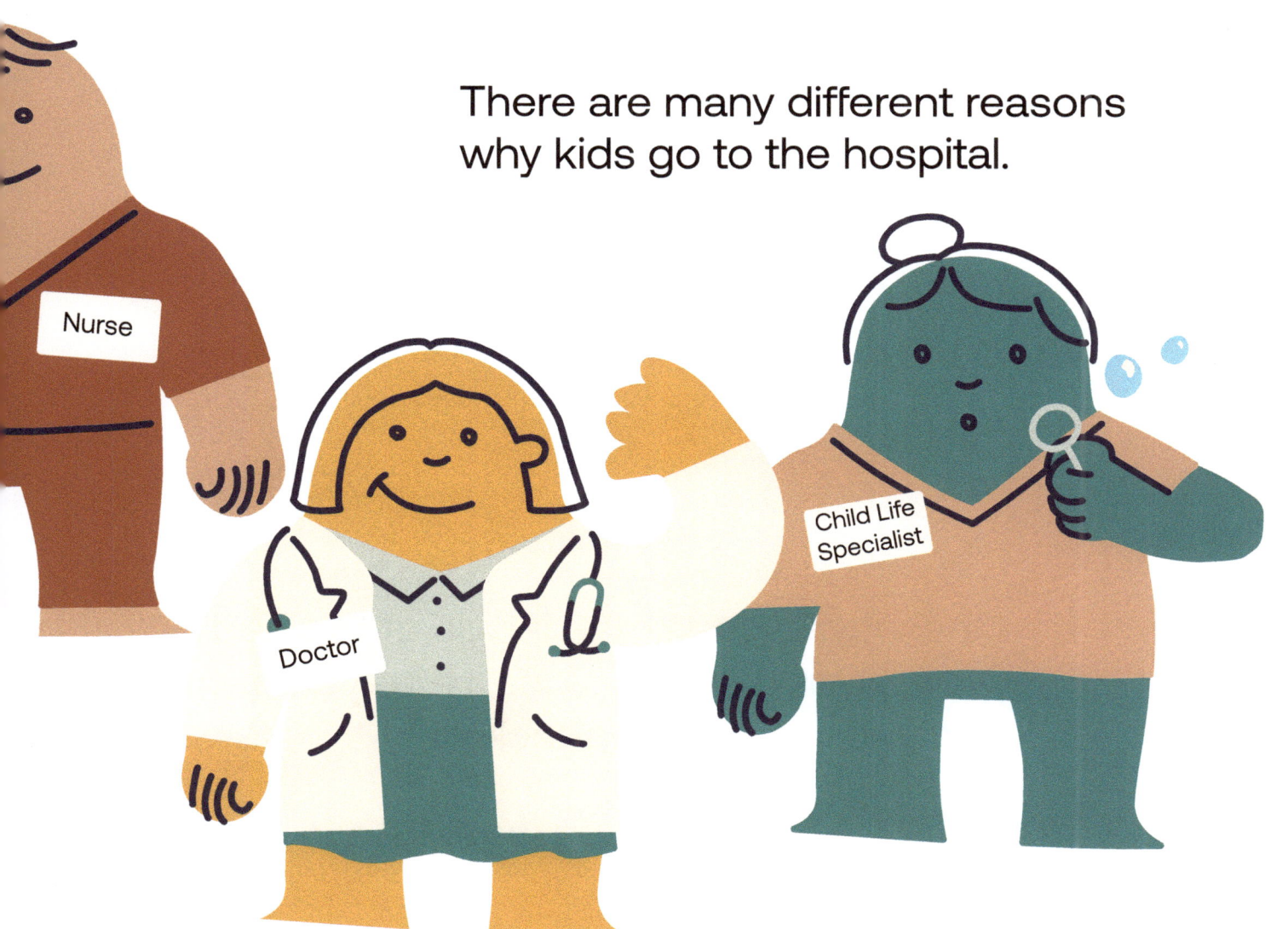

There are many different reasons why kids go to the hospital.

Sometimes, kids go to the hospital when their stomach hurts.

The team of doctors and nurses will gather more information about what is happening inside a kid's body, so they can make a plan to help them feel better.

One way to check the inside of the body is by looking at vital signs. Have you ever had your vital signs checked?

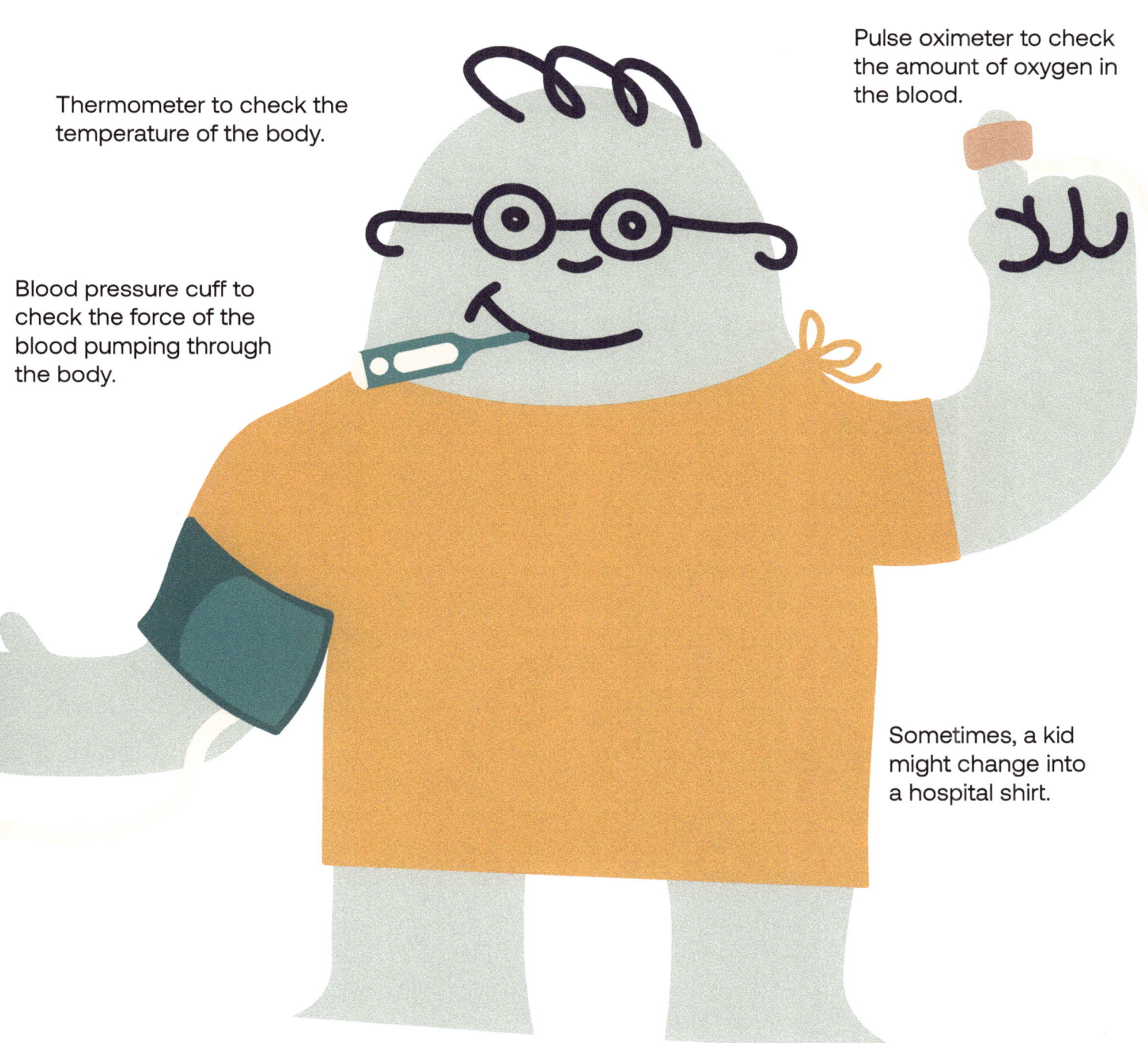

Thermometer to check the temperature of the body.

Pulse oximeter to check the amount of oxygen in the blood.

Blood pressure cuff to check the force of the blood pumping through the body.

Sometimes, a kid might change into a hospital shirt.

Another way the team can get more information is by taking pictures of the inside of the body.

In the hospital, there are different types of cameras that a doctor may use.

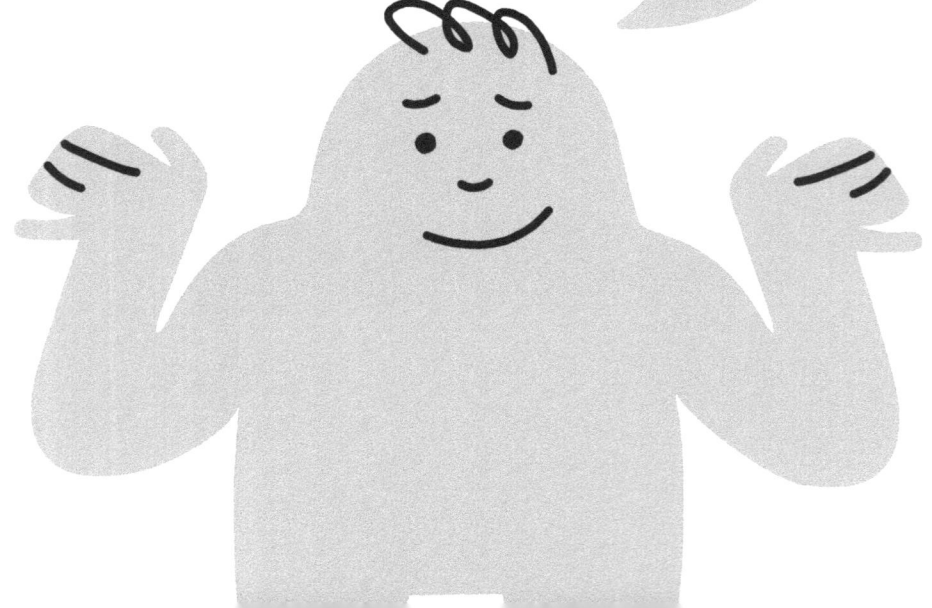

Does the camera go inside the body?

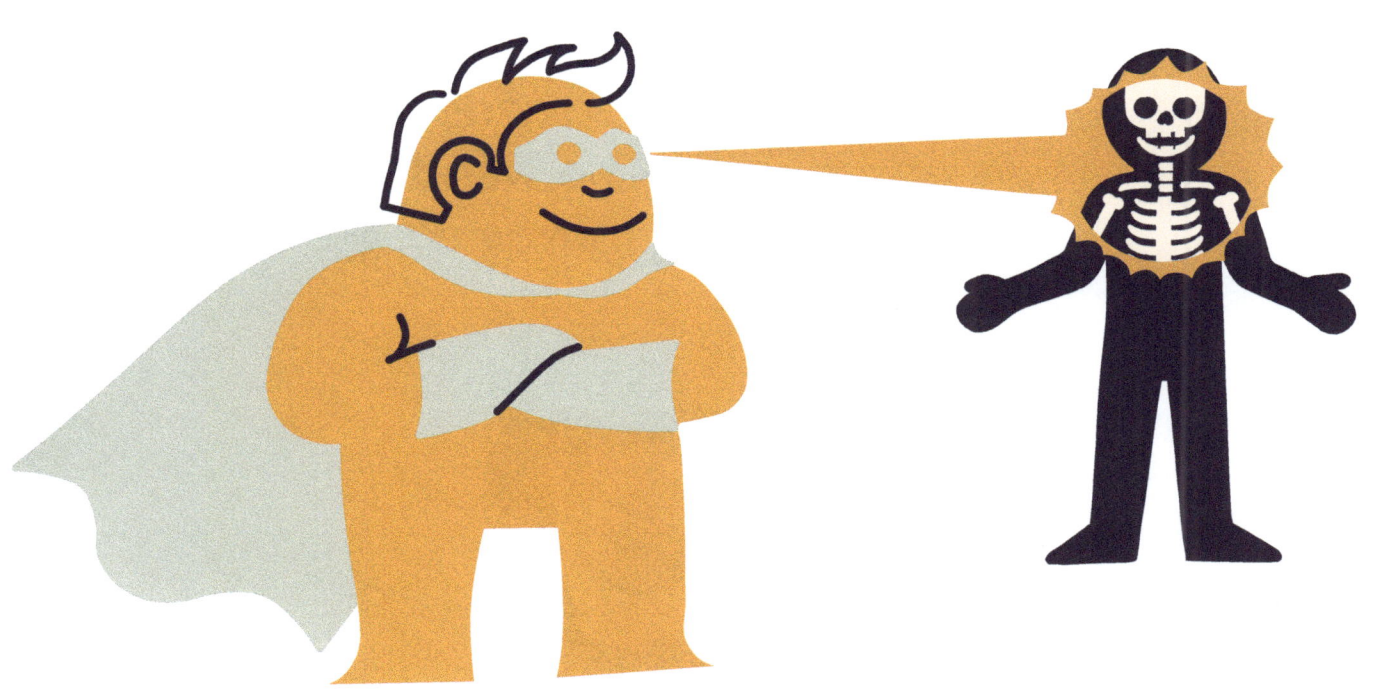

Nope, these specific cameras stay on the outside of the body but can see what is happening on the inside, like a superhero's x-ray vision.

One type of camera is called an ultrasound machine.

This machine is made up of a computer and a wand. The wand uses gel to take pictures as it moves across a kid's belly.

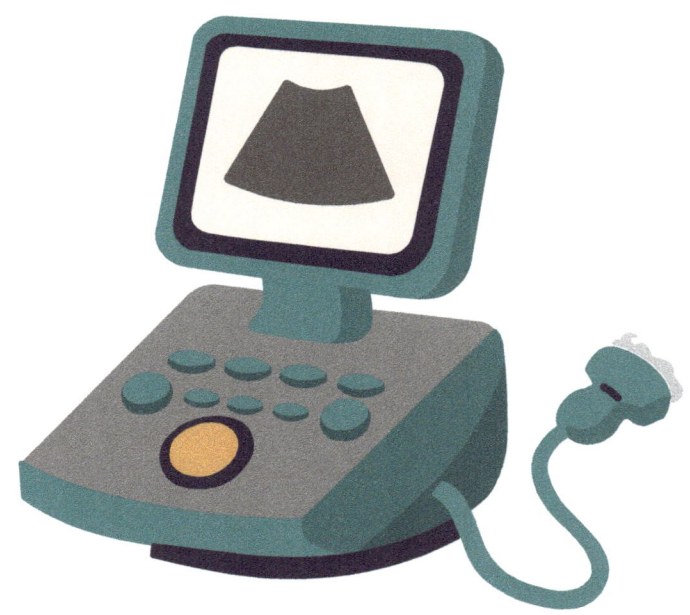

There are also other types of cameras doctors can use called CT (Computer Tomography) machines and MRI (Magnetic Resonance Imagining) machines.

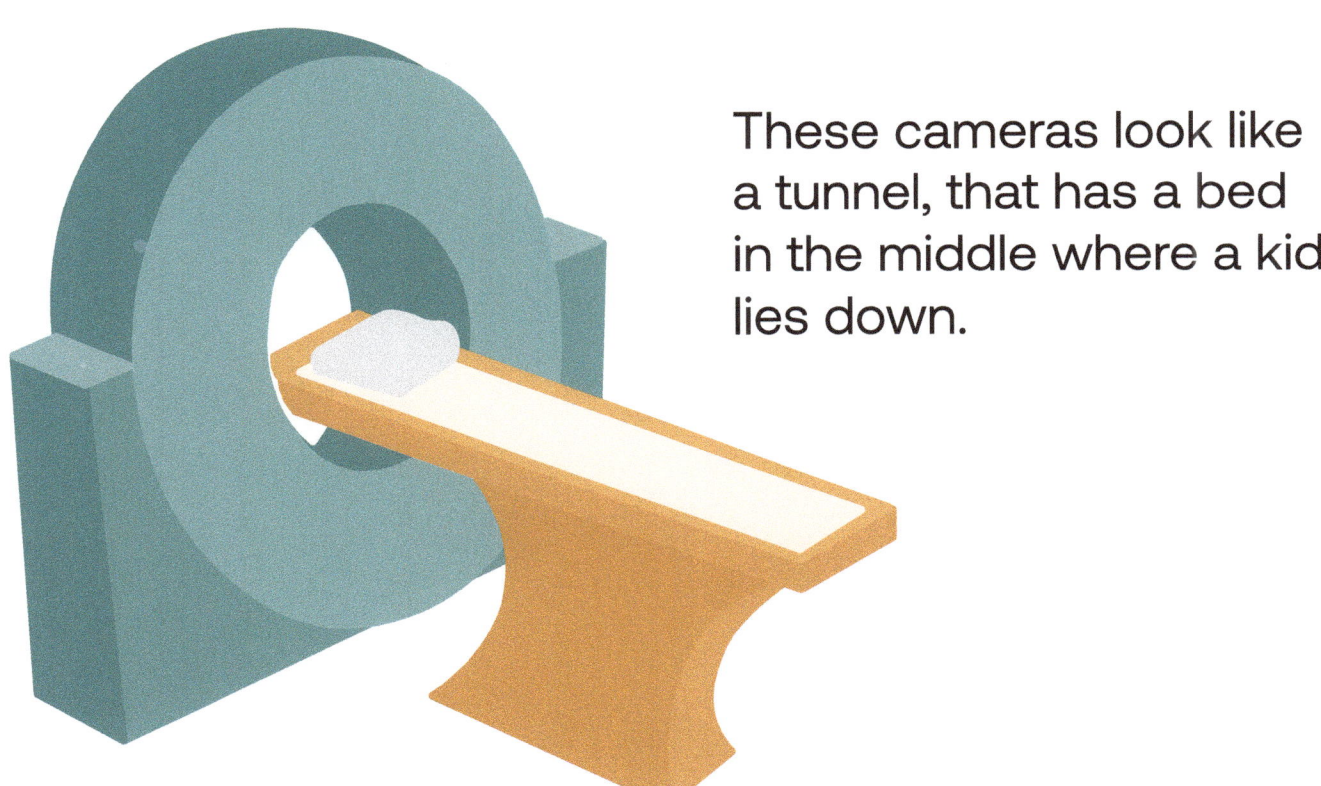

These cameras look like a tunnel, that has a bed in the middle where a kid lies down.

When the pictures are being taken, the bed slides in and out of the tunnel.

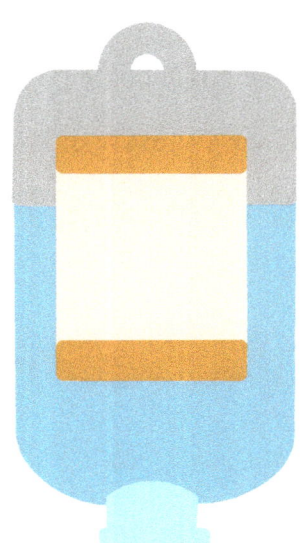

Doctors can also learn about what is happening inside a kid's body by checking their blood.

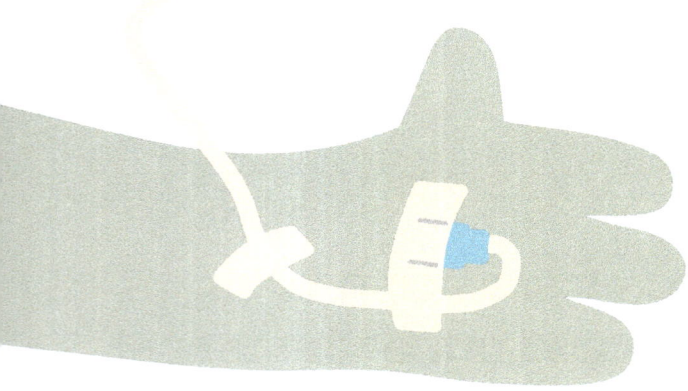

One way to check blood is through an IV (intravenous). An IV is a small, thin tube that connects to the inside of a kid's body.

It is also helpful to give a kid's body the water it needs and medicine to help if their stomach hurts.

Sometimes, the pictures and information show the doctors that a kid's tummy hurts because their appendix is sick.

If you're like me, you might be wondering what an appendix is and how did it get sick?

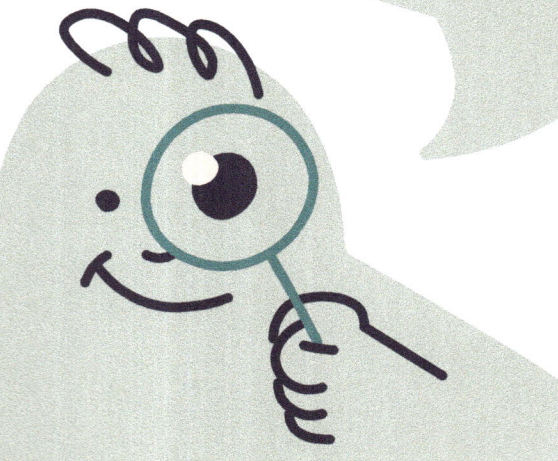

Well, the appendix is an organ or body part that is inside the body.

As far as doctors know, the appendix does not have a job like the heart or lungs do.

The appendix is a tube-shaped pouch that is attached to the intestines on the right side of the body.

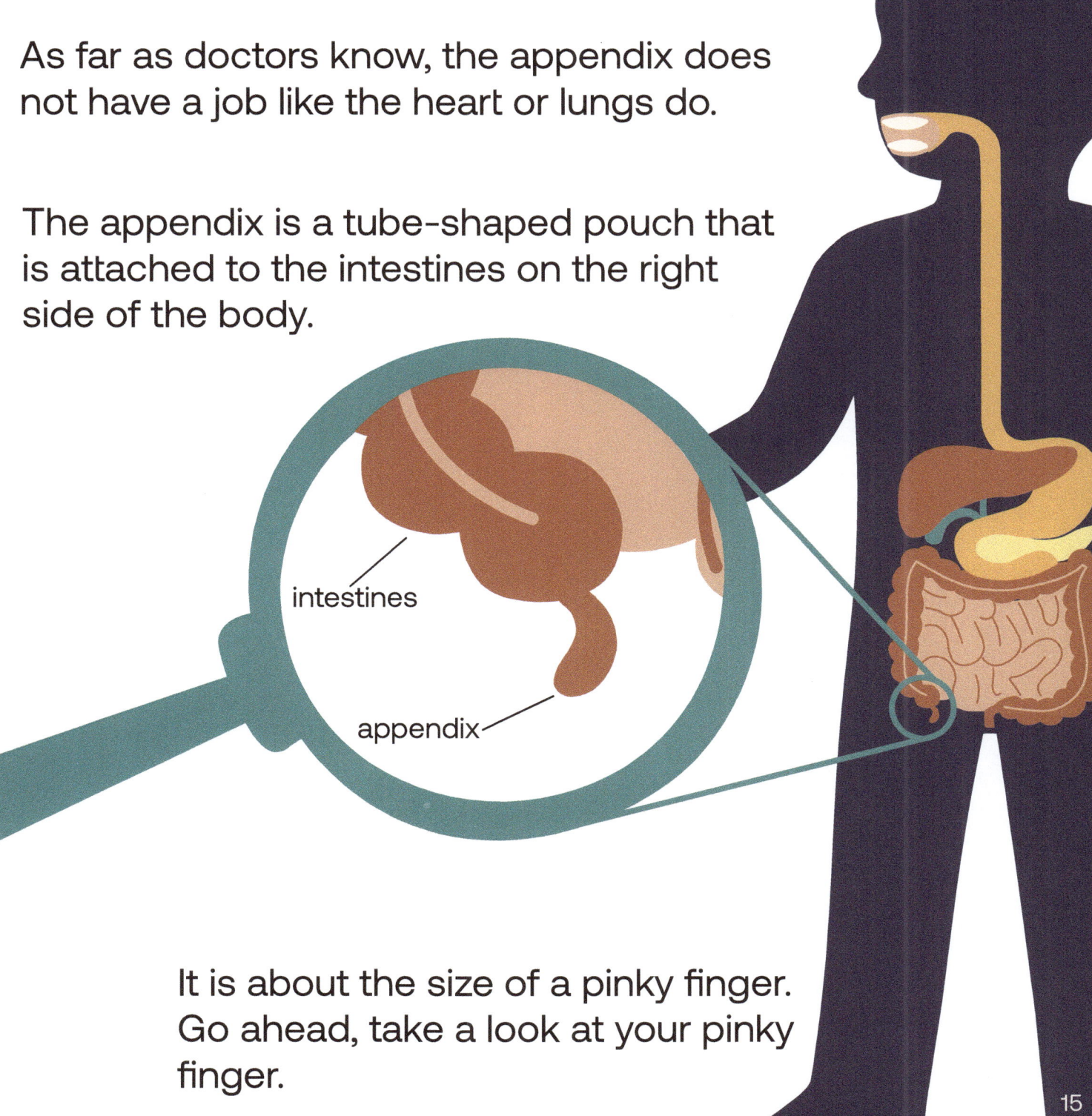

intestines

appendix

It is about the size of a pinky finger. Go ahead, take a look at your pinky finger.

When a kid's appendix gets sick,
it is called **appendicitis.**

This happens when there is a blockage where the appendix connects to the intestines.

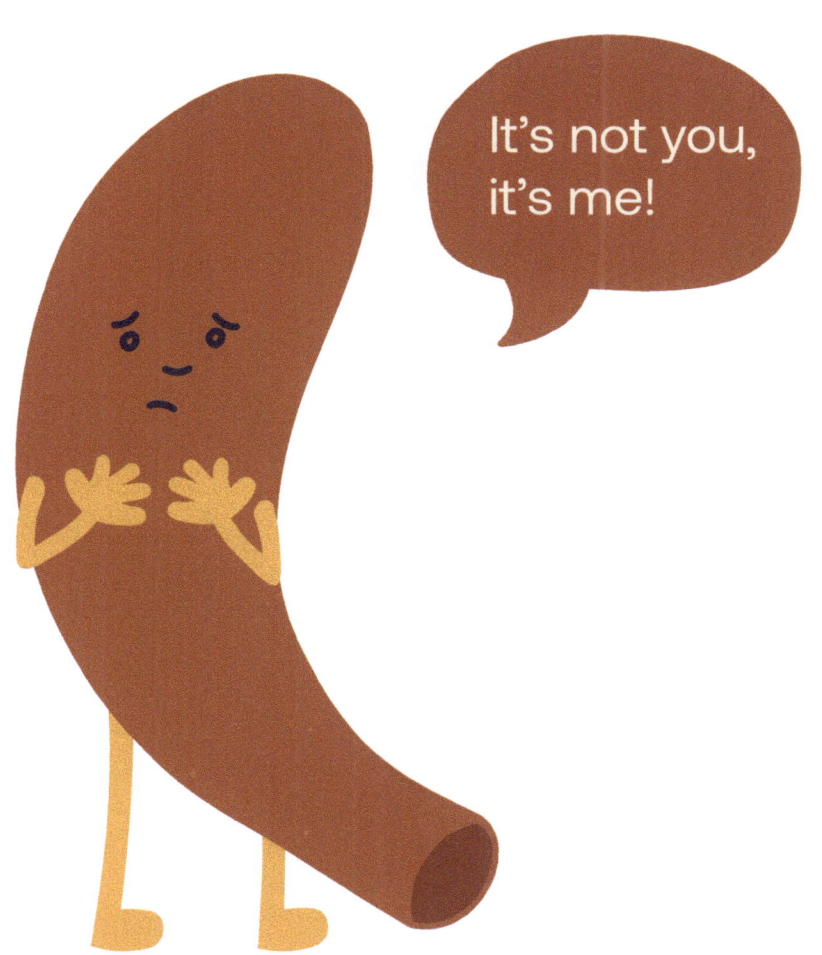

When there is a blockage, it can cause an infection inside the appendix. This makes the appendix inflamed or swollen.

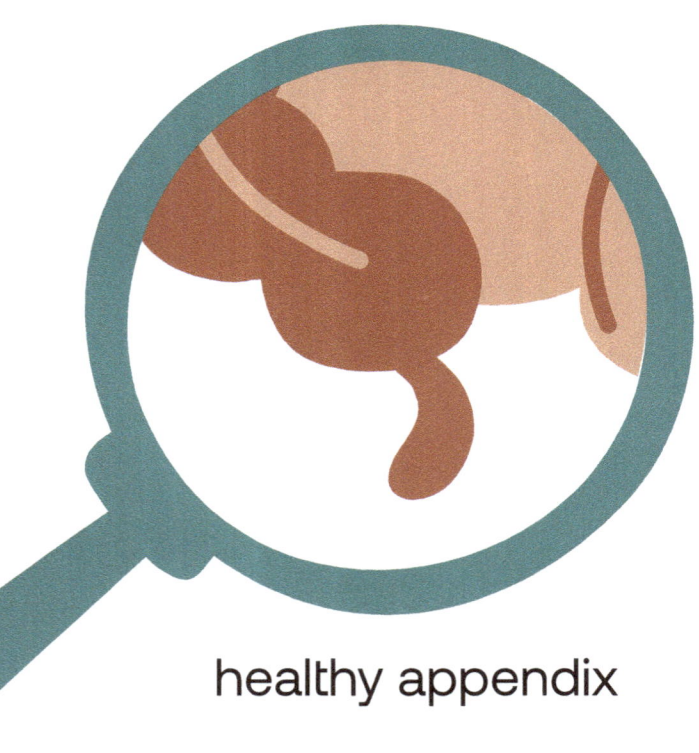

healthy appendix

appendicitis

Doctors do not know why some people get appendicitis and some people do not.

Appendicitis is no one's fault, no one can cause it to happen. Also, it is good to know appendicitis is not contagious, like a cold.

It is important to be in the hospital with appendicitis because it is the best place for doctors to help someone feel better.

A doctor can give a kid medicine to help their appendix feel better, or the appendix may need to be removed.

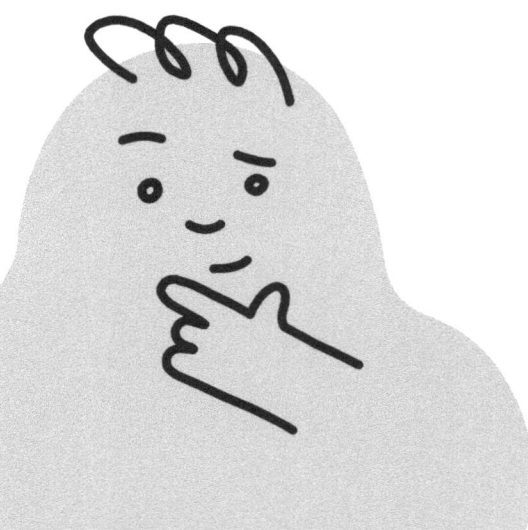

Whoa, what? Remove the appendix?

When a kid needs to have their appendix removed, they have something called **surgery.**

Surgery is when a doctor helps the inside of a kid's body.

Surgery to remove a kid's appendix is called an **appendectomy.**

There is another team of people whose entire job is to help a kid's body during surgery.

They wear matching clothes, hats, and masks to keep from sharing germs.

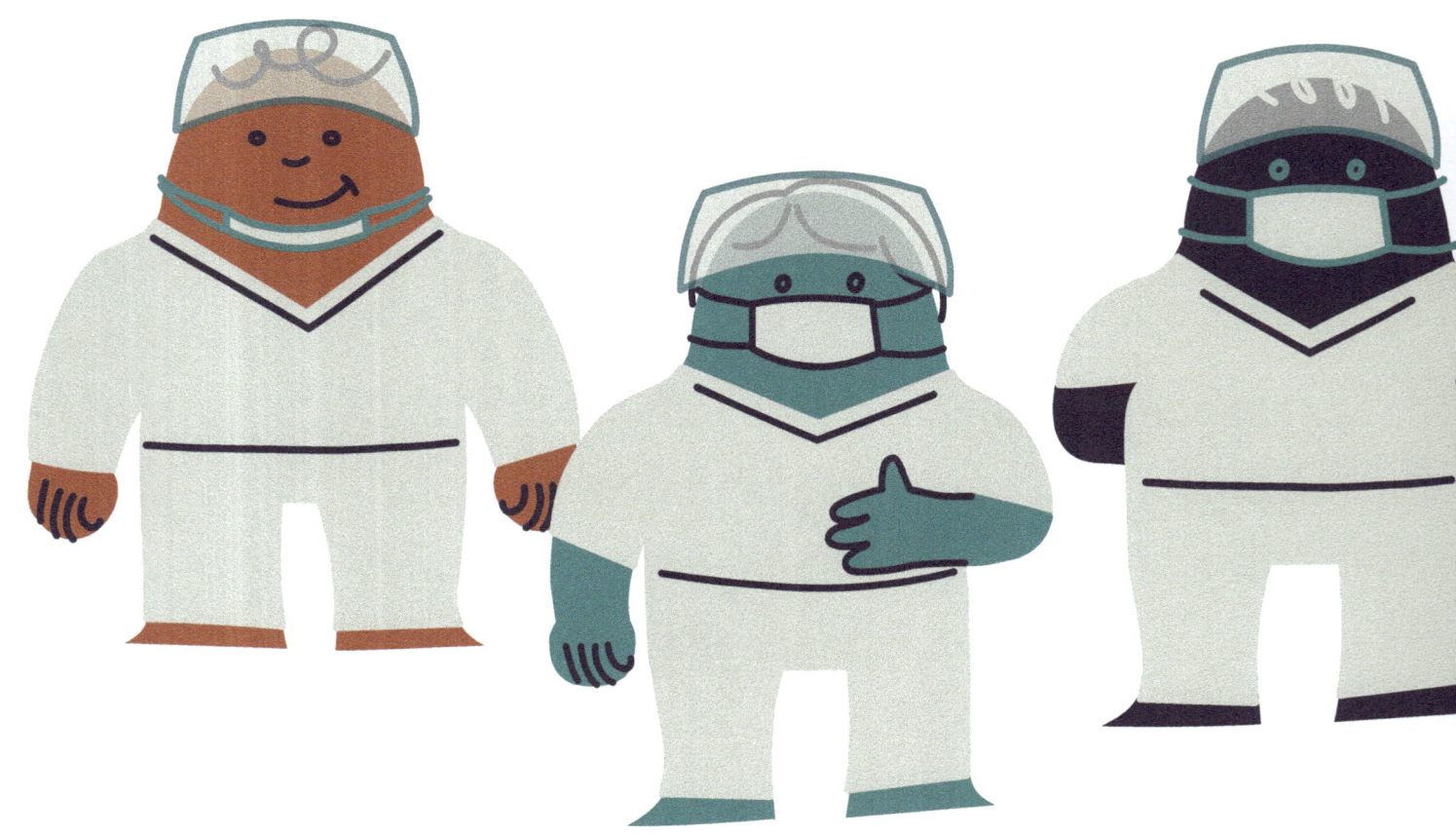

Surgery happens in a different room that is super clean.

This room might have a bed for a kid to sit up or lie down on, bright lights, and computer machines. All of these things help the doctors do their job during surgery.

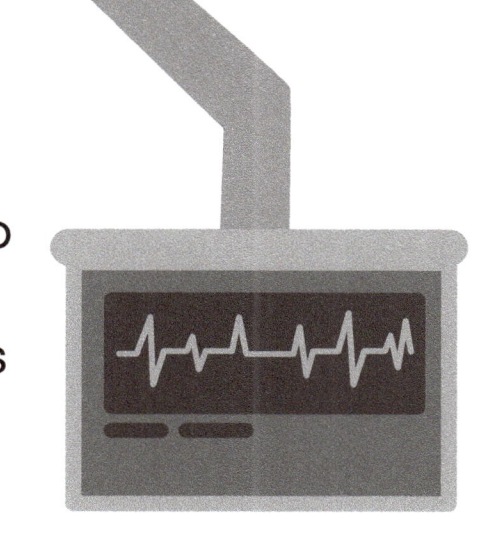

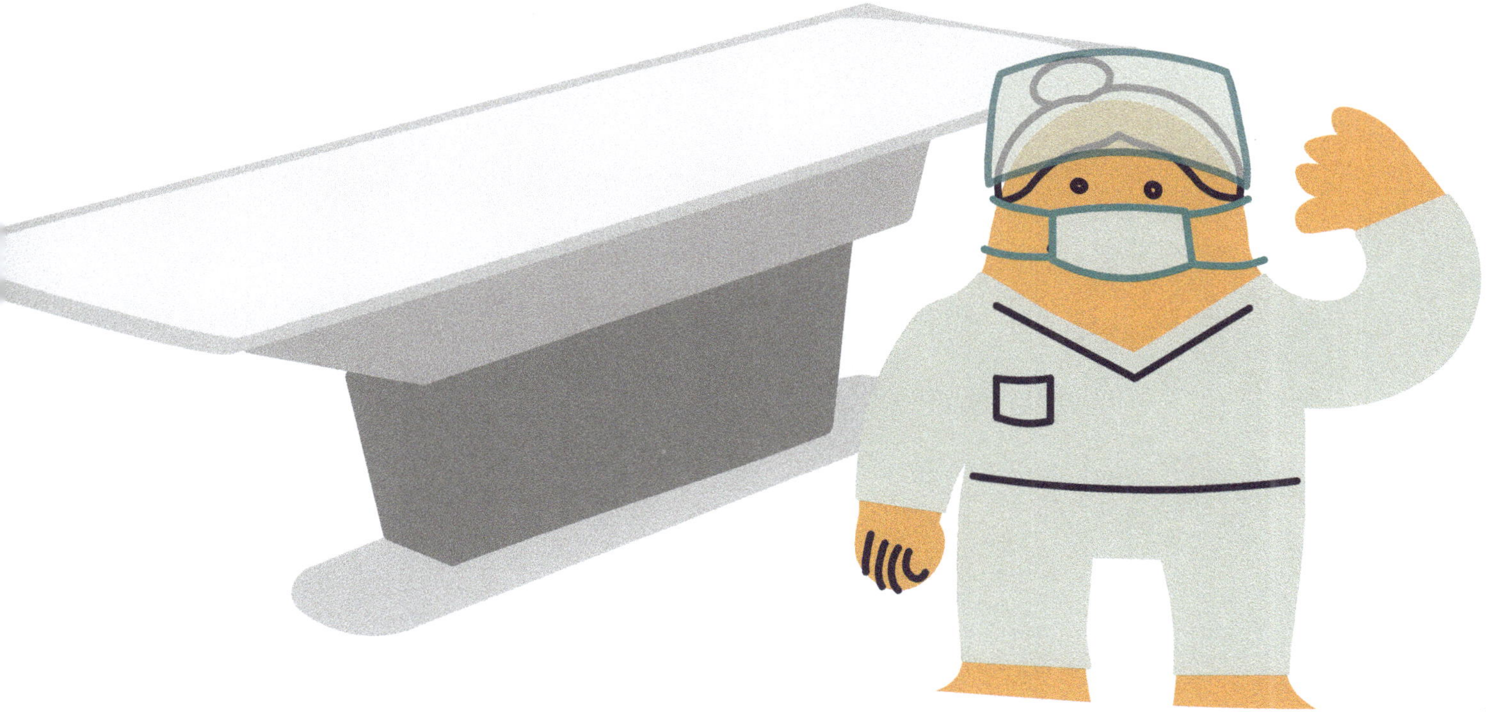

When a kid needs to have an appendectomy, they are given a medicine called

anesthesia

(sleeping medicine).

Anesthesia makes their whole body go to sleep so they will not feel, see, or hear anything.

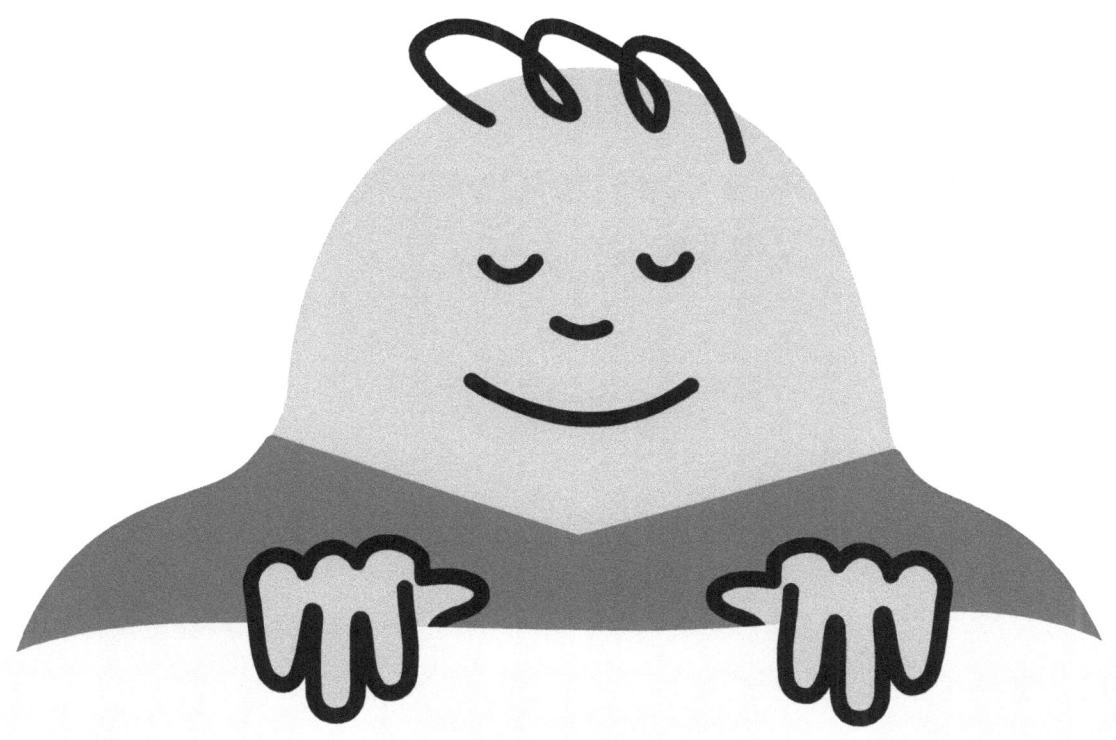

This kind of sleep is different than when someone goes to sleep on their own at night.

When the doctor stops giving the sleeping medicine, their body wakes up.

Anesthesia medicine can be given to a kid through their IV tube...

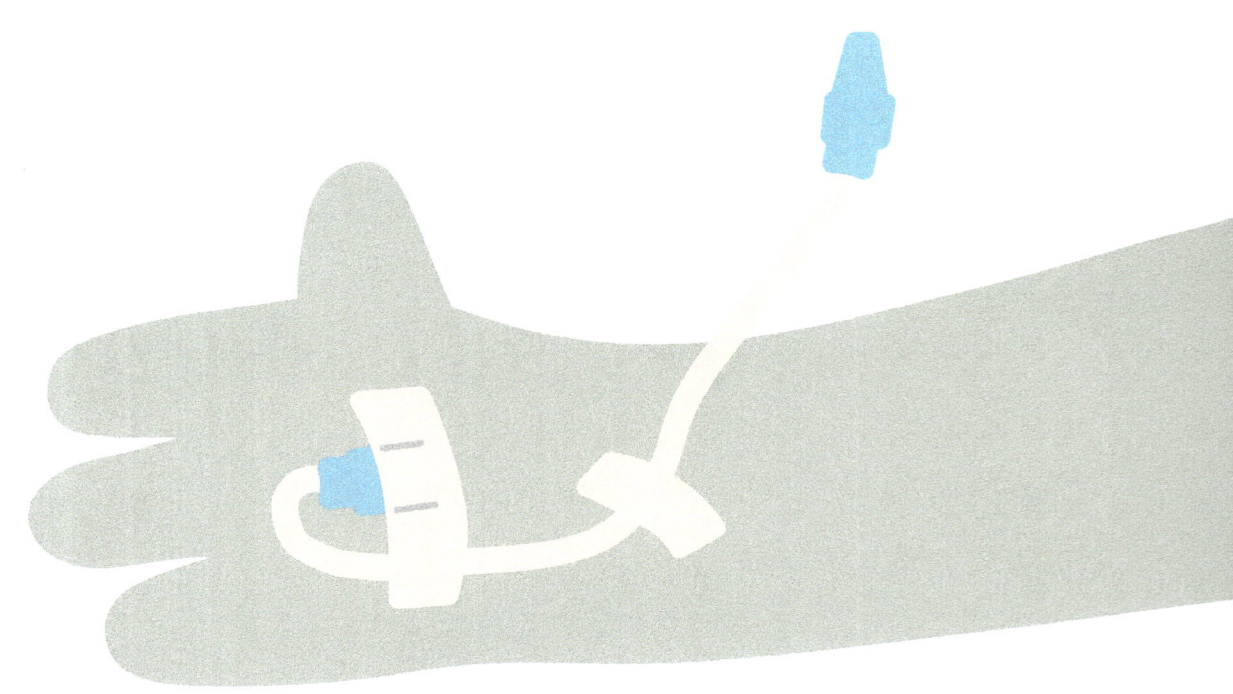

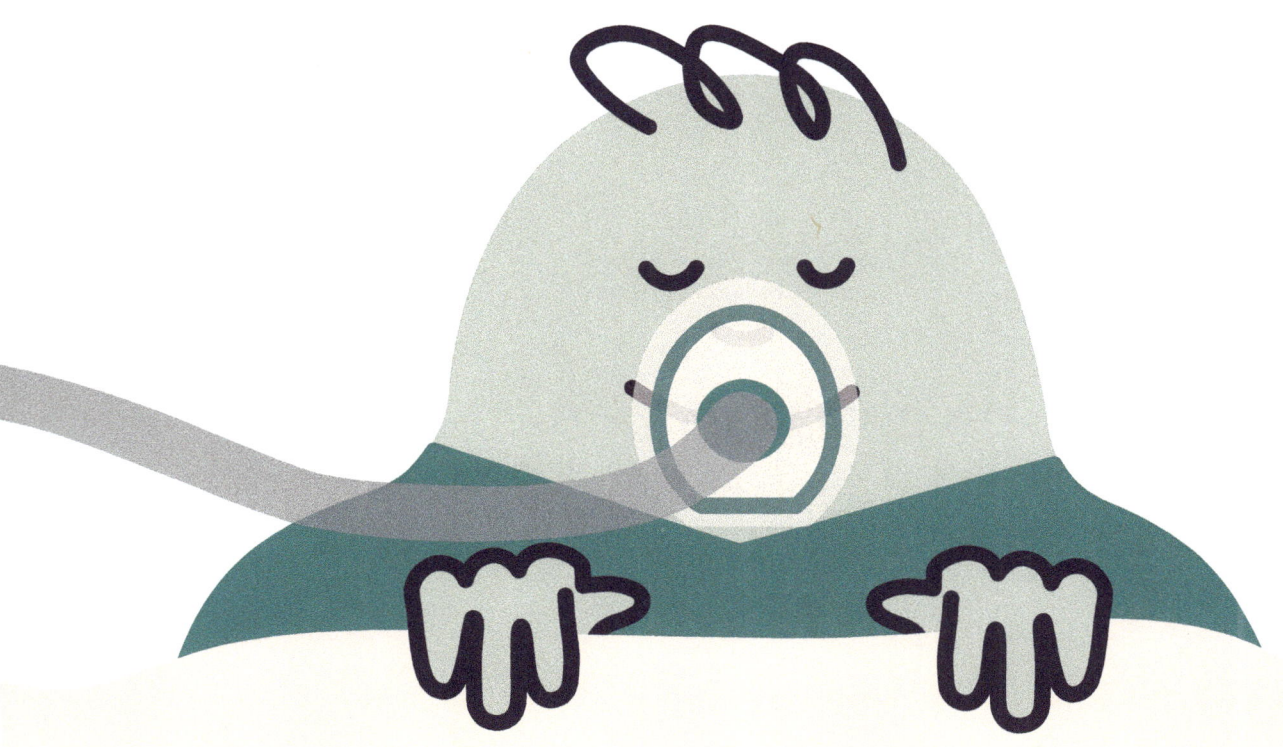

...Or through a mask where they breathe in the medicine.

Once a kid is given sleeping medicine and they are asleep, the doctors will disconnect and remove the appendix.

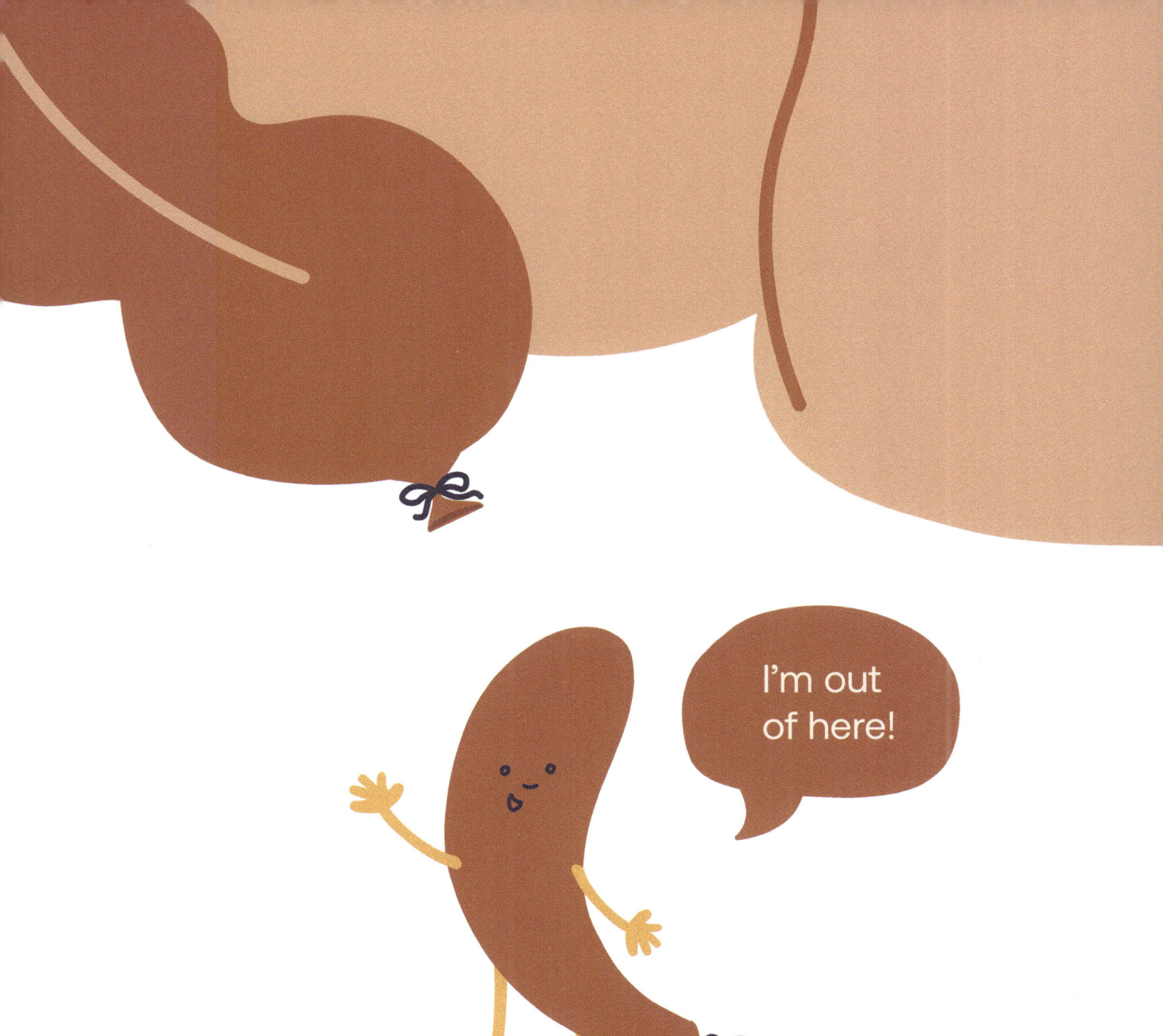

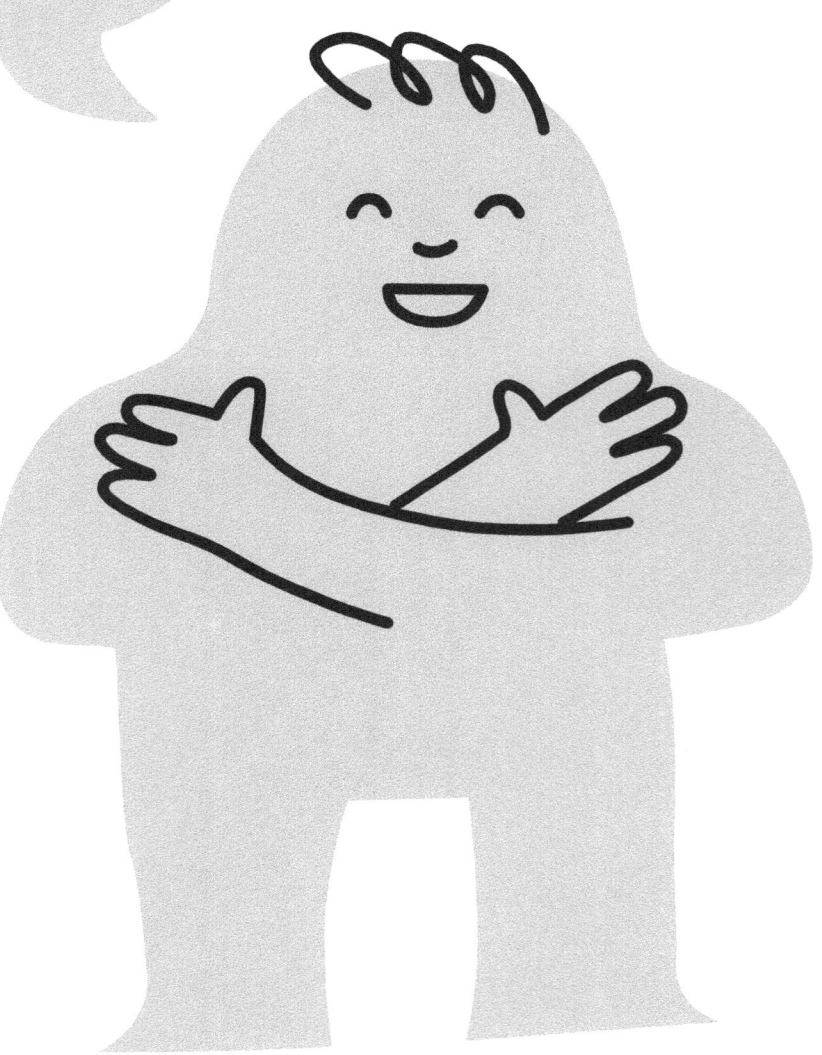

Remember, the appendix does not have a job, so a kid's body will work normally without their appendix.

There are lots of kids, teenagers, and adults who do not have their appendix and you would not even know.

After surgery, a kid will have some bandages on their belly.

It will be important for a kid to get up and walk around, eat or drink something, and let the doctors know how their body is feeling.

They might also have to stay overnight in the hospital until the doctors feel their body is ready to go home.

After a kid goes home, they will need to continue to let their body rest and heal.

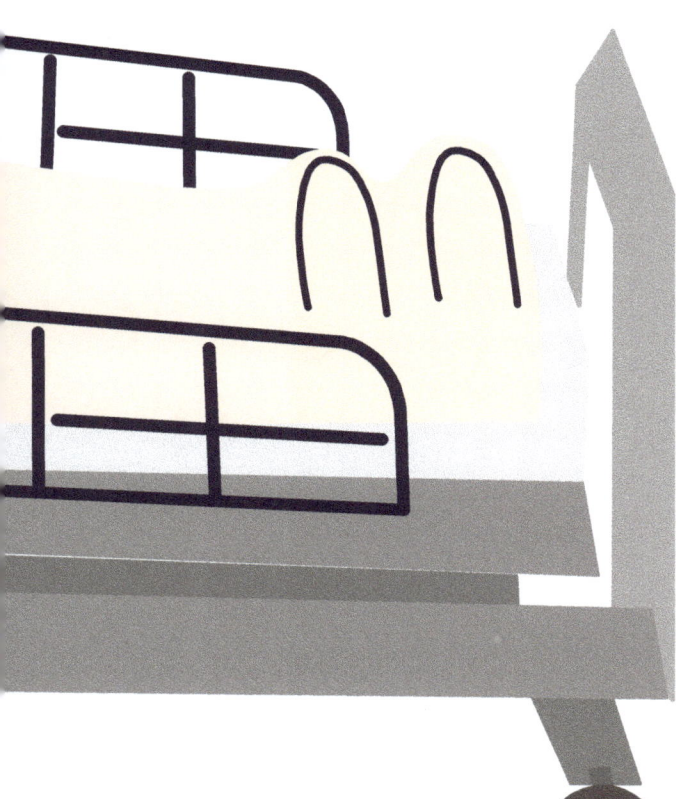

Soon they will be back doing all of the things they love to do.

Thanks for learning about the appendix and an appendectomy with us today.

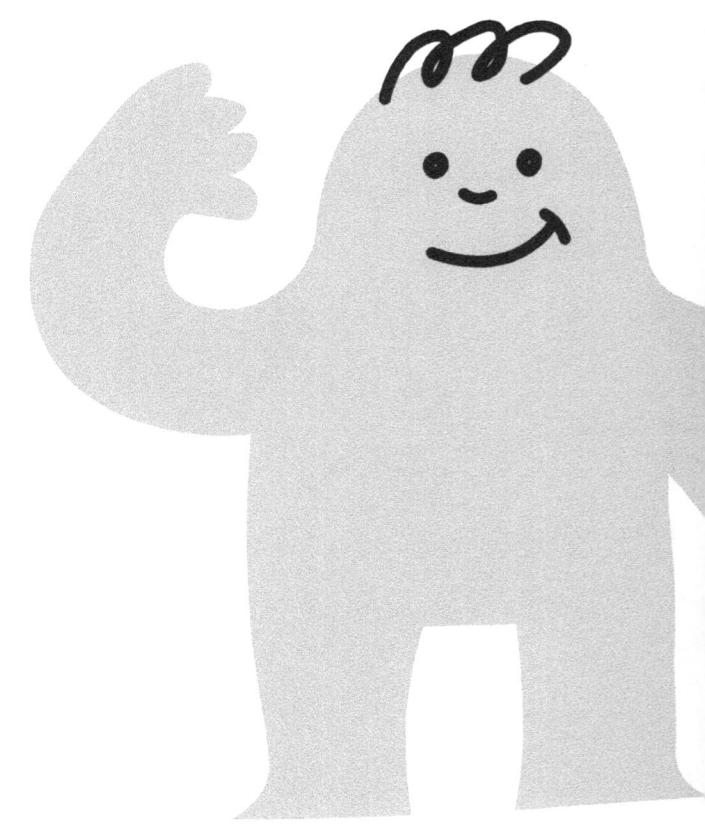

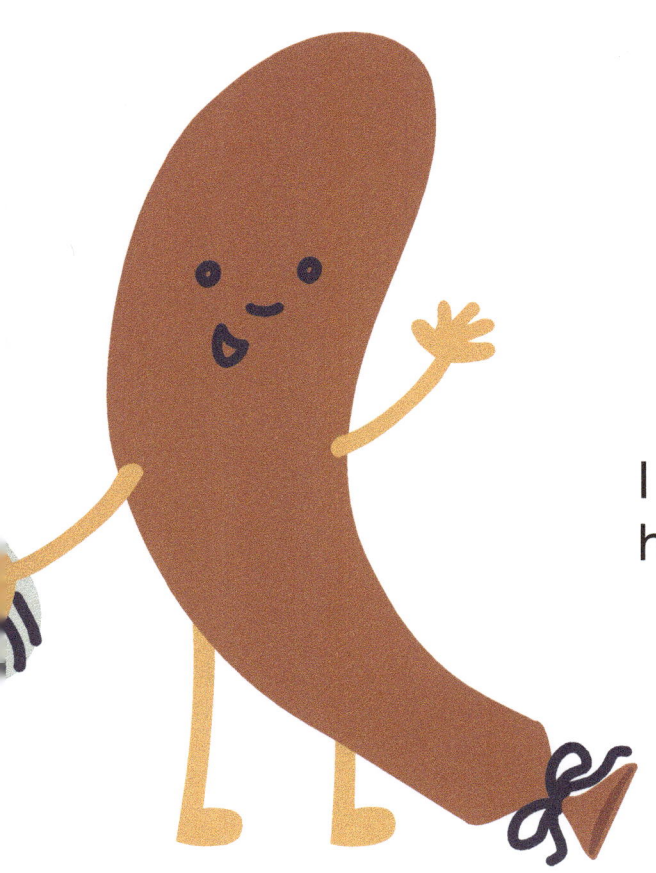

I wonder if you know anyone who has had their appendix removed?

Glossary

Anesthesia

When someone has surgery, they are given a medicine called anesthesia. Anesthesia makes their body go to sleep so they won't hear, see or feel anything. This kind of sleep is different than when someone goes to sleep on their own at night. When the doctor stops giving the sleepy medicine their body wakes up.

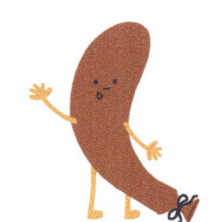

Appendectomy

An appendectomy is a surgery to disconnect and remove an appendix that is sick.

Appendicitis

Appendicitis is when there is a blockage where the appendix connects to the intestines. The blockage leads to an infection inside the appendix, causing the appendix to become inflamed and swollen. This can make a kid feel sick, nauseous, or make their stomach hurt.

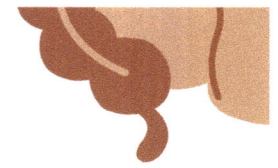

Appendix

The appendix is an organ inside the body. It is a tube-shaped pouch about the size of a pinky finger, attached to the intestines on the right side of the abdomen. As far as doctors know, the appendix does not have a job.

CT Scan (Computed Tomography)

A CT scan is one way to take pictures of the inside of a kid's body. A CT scan is a camera that looks like a tunnel with a bed in the middle where a kid lays down. When the pictures are being taken, the bed slides in and out of the tunnel.

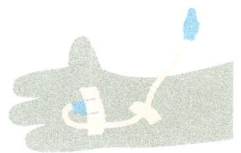

IV (Intravenous)

An IV is a small straw that goes into a vein. It can be used to check the blood and give a kid's body medicine or drinks of water.

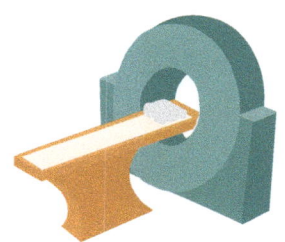

MRI (Magnetic Resonance Imaging)

An MRI scan is a way to take pictures of the inside of a kid's body. An MRI scan is a camera that looks like a tunnel with a bed in the middle where a kid lays down. When the pictures are being taken, the bed slides in and out of the tunnel.

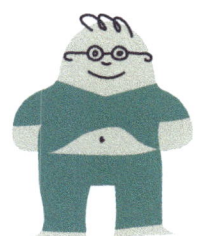

Surgery

Surgery is when a doctor helps the inside of someone's body.

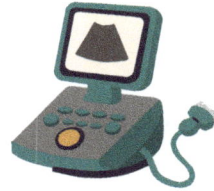

Ultrasound

Ultrasound is a machine to help collect information about what is happening inside of a kid's body by taking pictures. The machine is made up of a computer and a wand. The wand uses jelly to take pictures as it moves across a kid's belly.

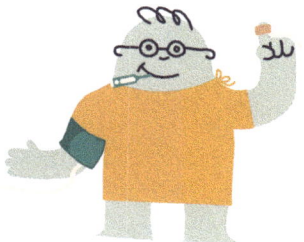

Vital Signs

Vital signs are a way doctors and nurses can gather information about what is happening inside a kid's body and how it is working. Vital sign information is gathered with a thermometer, a blood pressure cuff, and a pulse oximeter.

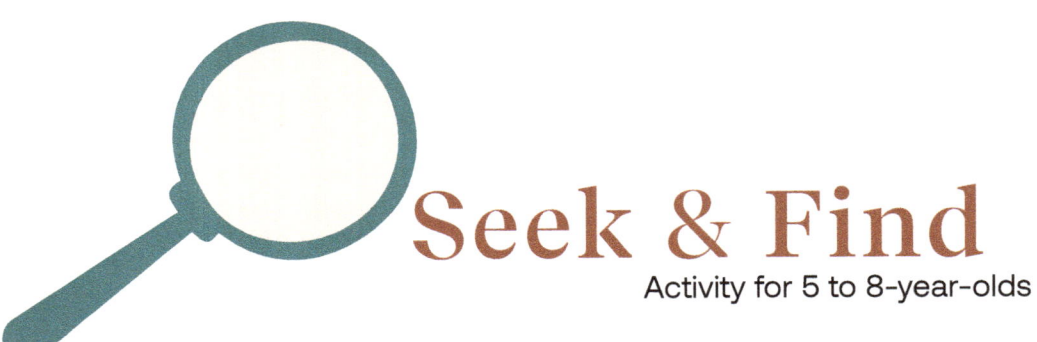

Seek & Find

Activity for 5 to 8-year-olds

Can you find and circle the images?

Camera with a computer and a wand that has gel on it.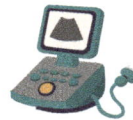

The organ in your body that is a tube-shaped pouch and has no job.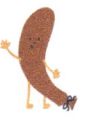

The tool that is like a band around the arm giving it a squeeze to check the force of the blood pumping through the body.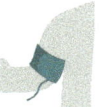

Find some team members who help someone's body feel better when they are at the hospital.

Someone getting the medicine that makes them go to sleep for surgery.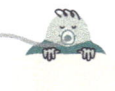

A small, bendy tube that connects to someone's body and can give them medicine.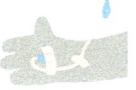

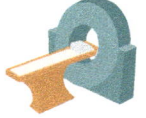

Camera with a tunnel and bed.

The tool that checks the temperature of the body.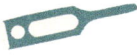

The tool that looks like a bandaid on a finger that checks how much oxygen is in someone's blood.

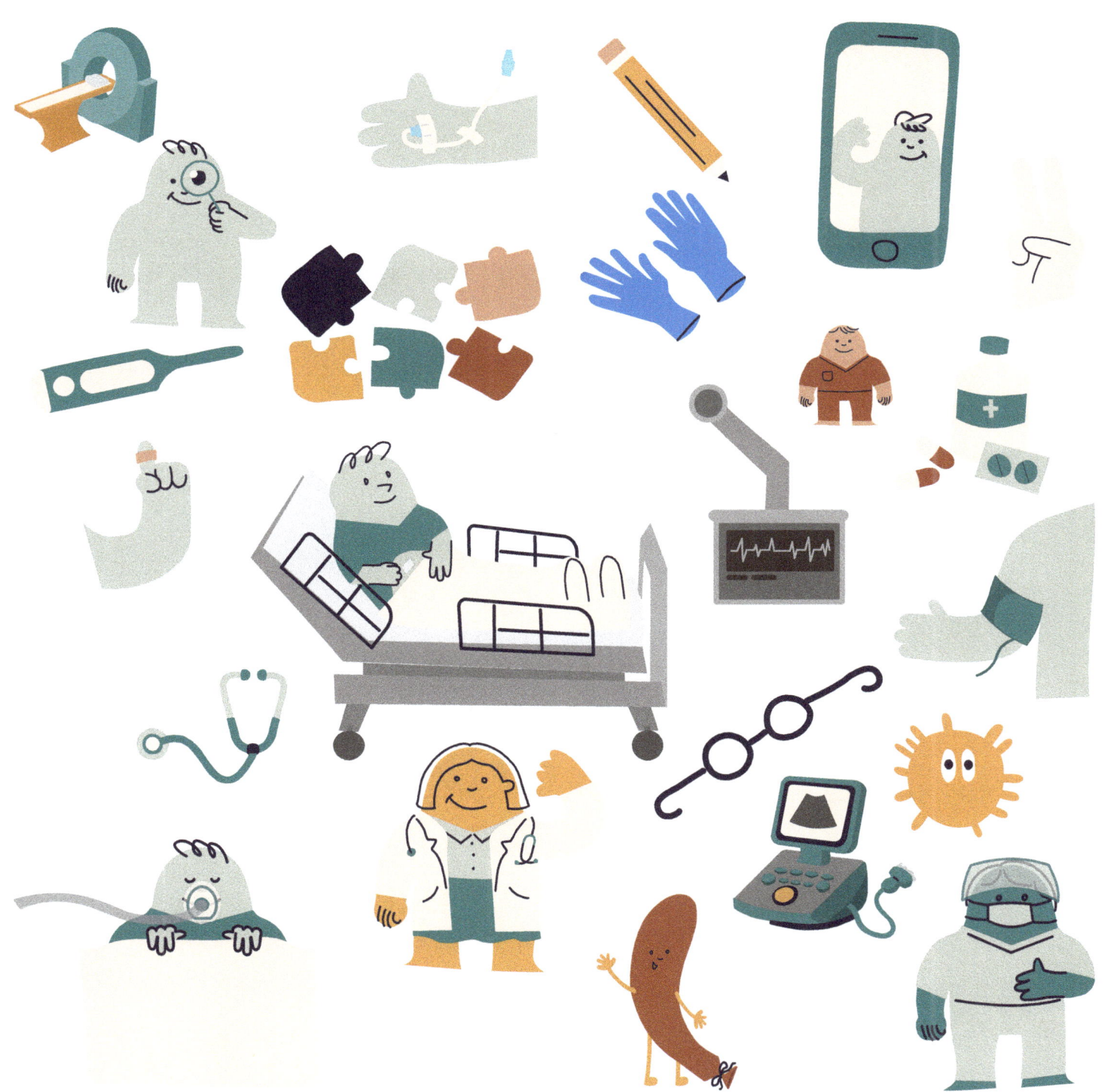

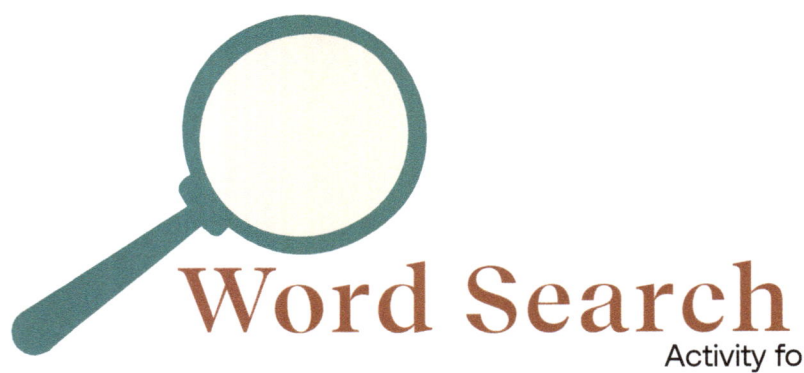

Word Search

Activity for 8 to 11-year-olds

Join your child in figuring out the answers and finding the words. Answers in the back.
***Bonus: Do you see any of these items in your room?**

The name of a scan where someone lays down on a bed that slides in and out of a tunnel.

The name of the scan that uses a wand and gel to take pictures.

The name of a small, bendy tube that connects to someone's body and can give them medicine.

The name of the organ in your body that is a tube-shaped pouch and has no job.

The tool that takes someone's temperature.

The name of the tool that checks how much oxygen is in someone's blood.

The name of the medicine that someone gets when they have surgery that makes them go to sleep.

The name of the surgery that someone might have when their appendix gets sick.

Two team members who help someone's body feel better when they are at the hospital.

*QR Code for answer key on next page

```
H A M A U K E Q O W B I
Z Z T P L C D P M A Y A
D V H P T Z F U T B K N
O T E E R P S L A N W E
C Y R N A V O S P U N S
T C M D S P Y E P R I T
O B O E O Z S O E S L H
R X M C U M W X N E R E
Q W E T N I G C D P Y S
X I T O D T Z A I Y P I
J I E M Y M R I X I P A
Z T R Y S I C L H N V X
```

Scan the QR code for more information about how to prepare and support your child.

Scan with your phone's camera here!

Find the word search answer key on our website here!

Text copyright © 2025 Child Core Family Support LLC.

All rights reserved.

No part of this book may be reproduced or transmitted in any form or by any means, electronic or mechanical, including photocopying, recording, or by any information storage and retrieval system, without written permission from the publisher.

The only exception is brief quotations for reviews.

For information please contact author at hello@childcorefamilysupport.com

ISBN: 979-8-9987553-4-7

The information in this book is based on our own education, research, and experience. It is designed to be used as a tool to support a child's understanding of the topic of an appendectomy and not in lieu of already existing supports, consults, or medical information provided by Child Life Specialists or other medical professionals.

For more information about Child Life Specialists and how they can help, go to childcorefamilysupport.com.

Written by: Madison Matthews, B.S., CCLS, Caitlin McNamara, M.S., CCLS, CIMI & Adrienne O'Connor, M.S., CCLS
Illustrated by: Adrienne O'Connor, MS, CCLS

www.ingramcontent.com/pod-product-compliance
Lightning Source LLC
Chambersburg PA
CBHW040005040426
42337CB00033B/5232